FOCUS YOUR FIGURE

Also by Toni Beck and Patsy Swank

Fashion Your Figure: The Ten-Minutes-a-Day Program for Fitness

FOCUS YOUR FIGURE

A PERSONAL PROGRAM FOR NATURAL EXERCISE

BY TONI BECK AND PATSY SWANK

Illustrated by GEORGE EISENBERG

1973
HOUGHTON MIFFLIN COMPANY BOSTON

CONTENTS

A portion of this book has appeared in *McCall's*.

First Printing   H

ISBN: 0–395–13946–5
Library of Congress Catalog Card Number: 72–514
Printed in the United States of America

INTRO-
DUCTION

With our first book, *Fashion Your Figure*, we proposed to you a program of exercise which you could adapt to your own needs, rather than a torture rack on which to hang yourself.

We think that beautiful movement is an important element in every woman's life, but that, for one reason or another, many women miss the beauty and health rewards it provides and the simple sensuous satisfaction that it gives. Exercise is the door that leads to that satisfaction.

We do not think, however, that every woman requires the same kind of exercise or the same amount. What is more, she will gain most from a program which she can adapt to her own goals, provided — and these are important provisions — she can be helped to ascertain reasoned and valid goals and is given a range of alternative choices in which she has complete confidence.

The range we offer comes from the exercise program which Toni Beck evolved (from her own system) especially for use at the Greenhouse, a beauty retreat between Dallas and Fort Worth which is operated by the Great Southwest Corporation with the guidance of Charles of the Ritz and the Neiman-Marcus Company. All of these exercises have been found directly and repeatedly effective during six years of intensive work with women of all ages, temperaments, and constitutions.

Fashion Your Figure offered a basic overall pro-

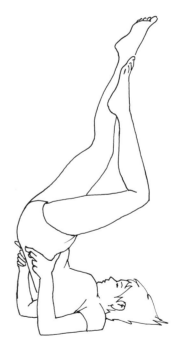

gram which required ten minutes a day of its users and provided extensions of the basic movements for more intensive work or attack on problem areas.

Focus Your Figure may be called a magnifier, for we will start at the head and work to the feet, dividing the body into general areas with a chapter on each. In each of these chapters will be specific single exercises, then groupings of them (or *enchaînements,* as the ballet people say) that incorporate the whole subject area, and finally a section on pertinent exercises (The Throwaways) you can do while you are supposed to be doing something else (or Anything to Get Exercise off the Pad).

Some of them seem similar and are not (i.e., a raised palm turned out has a different effect on the inner arm from a raised palm turned in). Some seem similar and are, because very slight variations sometimes make an exercise easier for one person than another without changing what is to be achieved.

You will find repetition of points we consider vital — breathing, posture, pelvic position. Whatever emphasis we figure will help you remember, we use!

These exercises can of course serve in a reducing program, as they do at the Greenhouse, but the book is not designed primarily as a reducing manual. Use it, at first, to burn up unwanted calories, but get past that stage as expediently as you can and once you have evolved your personal style (not the one fashion dictates, nor your children, nor even your favorite man, although he will probably have more to do with it than anyone), then fashion yourself an exercise program to keep it. Maybe more than one — maybe a few minutes of movement to wake up by, or to prepare yourself for sleep, or even a How-Did-I-Get-Myself-in-This-Nervous-Box one, or a Just-After-Christmas one. But enjoy the movement and make it beautiful — whether it is a noontime stretch, a water jog, or a bicycle kick to attack an abundant tummy. Remember, it is what will get you where you are going.

Toni Beck
Patsy Swank

CHAPTER 1

START WHERE YOU ARE—
RESTATEMENT OF PHILOSOPHY

The trouble with writing about exercises for specific body problems is that you run headlong into the Band-Aid or Cure-Me-Quick Syndrome. You become the one who says, "I can plug up this hole," and then watches the whole boat sink!

Therapists use isolated exercises to achieve certain things, but they use them within an overall framework of exercise. That is the way we hope that you will use those which follow. You can turn right away to the ones which will help you firm your arms or flatten your tummy — they are there. But if you use a good exercise program in such a confined context, or only to lose weight, you deny yourself the greatest part of its value. It is as if you took only enough to make a handkerchief from a beautiful yardage that could supply a whole dress.

We think you should feel that exercise is a vital part of the rhythm of your life. A rhythm which, for most people, is being increasingly obstructed by stress. It would seem, with all the beat going on around us, that rhythm would be no problem. The hang-up is overabundance. There is too much sound going in too many directions. There are so many different drummers to listen to. All this obscures your ability to listen to your own. These warring dynamics, if you want to be philosophical, form the pattern of your life — its peaks, its depths, its anticipations, and its boredoms. You have to learn to manage all of them.

If you want to be simplistic, you can say the

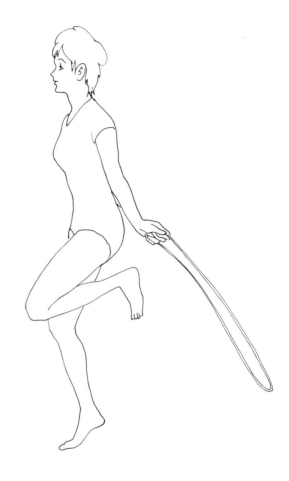

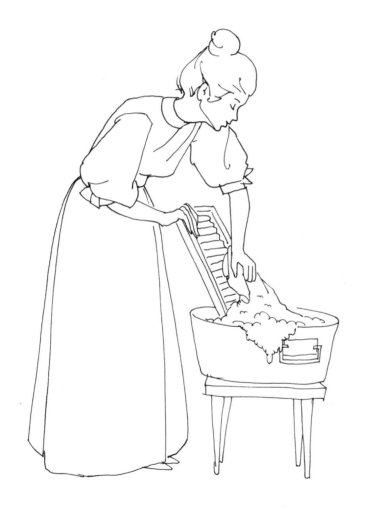

rhythm of your life is your heartbeat and your breath. But there is no denying that philosophy and physical fact are tied together, and so one of the important functions of a thoughtful exercise is to provide a kind of bottom rhythm for your life.

Long ago, that kind of rhythmic exercise was supplied by the difficulties of survival — chopping and hacking and scrubbing and rocking and running and hiding. Such a rhythm goes far toward keeping outside things in proper perspective. It still does, for the people who do it, but every generation has done it progressively less, and every generation seems to be in greater need of supplementing its vast mental and material achievements with the kind of simple body action that keeps everything in focus.

A part of the force behind the environmental movement is a desire to return to the untroubled beat of nature and to preserve a world where the natural cycles and processes will not be mutated by the crunch we sometimes call progress.

We have said before that one of the most important aspects of well-being is knowing yourself, and we have also admitted that this involves a good deal more than saying "Hello" as you pass a mirror. Can you, in sixty seconds, describe any specific rhythmic discipline in your life which would help you pace your health activities, improve your looks, serve, in fact, as a home base for your whole equilibrium?

A good exercise program can do that.

We trust you will understand that any such program must be accompanied by a course of sensible nutrition and reasonable rest, and we think anything you evolve for yourself should have the approval of your doctor. This does not mean a crash diet, or going to bed every night after the ten o'clock news. It does mean that you cannot take the program at full gallop. None of these exercises will harm the normal body, and virtually all of them can be adapted for special problems. If you have these, all the more reason to let your doctor check the program you evolve for yourself. He will tell you if there is a special kind of movement you should avoid. He will also, we trust, add a cheer for your good intentions.

Your heartbeat is the pulse of your life, but when you add everything up, the heart depends on the breath you send in. The whole mechanism, and the way it functions, is a miracle — not only physically but mentally. Breathing is the great air cushion. Properly done, it can get you wound up to great achievement and relax you from great effort. Unfortunately, we breathe less well all the time.

Because we have been provided with a splendid apparatus that gets the air in and out, most of us think we know how to breathe. What we know how to do is keep from suffocating, but as to giving a care about getting the breath well down into the lungs where it can work effectively, or toning the

3

muscles that handle the air traffic — well, we don't.

Breathing is the absolute cornerstone of any exercise program, but it might well be called the Forgotten Foundation. It is there. It happens. It will do so much for you only if you know how to use it.

The basic general rule for breathing in terms of exercise is that you breathe in when you are in stress (or when you are asking your muscles to work) and you exhale when you relax (or let your body rest). You will find that this fits very comfortably into most any body movement. If you do something that calls for raising an arm or lifting a leg, then you get your breath on the lift, let it out on the release. Inhale-exhale. Stress-release. In-out. Tense-relax.

The pattern is easy but not infallible. For instance, we typically hold our breath when we are trying to achieve something important to us, even in so basic a field as exercise. Therefore, you must accustom yourself to think of breathing itself as an exercise — which indeed it has been for many peoples for hundreds of years.

The threat of environmental pollution has made us acutely conscious of the importance of the kind of air we need. But we do not use to its full capacity the air we have.

In this context of physical and environmental consciousness, open your window (no matter how ridiculous it seems) and breathe deeply in front of it. You may leave it open while you do these exercises, unless the smog gets to you. That may suggest a different form of action.

Try these exercises.

1. Standing in good posture, clasp hands lightly in front of your chest. Slowly but steadily, breathe in; at the same time, turn the palms out and stretch arms up over the head. Stay in the stretch and hold your breath as long as it is comfortable. Then let the breath out slowly, loosen your hands, let the upper body collapse into a slump. Shake your hands and arms when they get back down to your side. Ten times.

2. Standing in good posture, pelvis tucked, hug yourself fondly with your palms at the back of your shoulders. Now breathe in slowly and when you have all you can hold, open your arms out to a wide Welcome-the-Day spread. Let your breath out as you gather your arms back into the hug.

Variation: Open your arms as you come to breath capacity and bend forward at the waist, back straight and arms out to the side in the spread. As you release breath slowly, gather the arms back, tuck the pelvis in, and roll the back, vertebra by vertebra, to the upright position of the hug. Eight times.

3. Tailor-sit with hands on the floor, backs down,

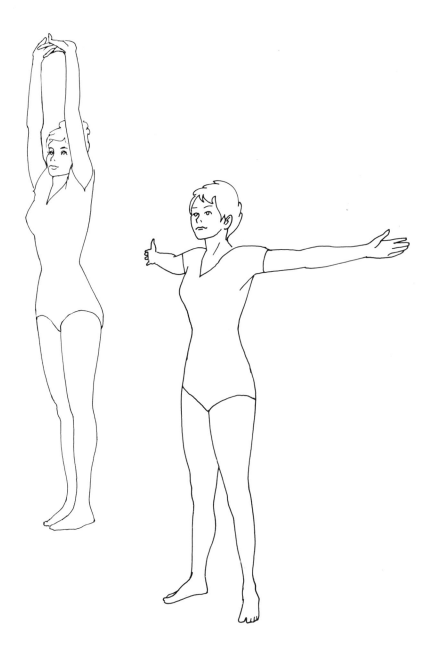

5

and slightly behind you. Relax the body forward, letting the head drop down to the floor if possible. Stay down as long as it is comfortable. Now breathe in and curl spine up to the straight position. Repeat, pressing air out of the body as it goes down. Eight times.

4. This is for presleep. In bed, lying on your back, knees bent, and feet flat. Breathe in, bring your legs up to your chest, and grasp them with your arms. Slowly let breath out, let knees relax, and drop back to starting position. Arms open to sides. Eight times.

CHAPTER 2

AN EXERCISE ROAD MAP—
HOW TO GO

Even after you establish a consciousness of breathing and coordinating it with a particular exercise, it is sometimes easy to get off beat or to forget, especially if you are tired or distracted when you begin. Because this happens to all of us, we suggest that when you work out your schedule, as the next chapter outlines, you take two or three full breaths before you start each group of the same exercises.

If you can think of anything we have forgotten to keep breath in the forefront of your mind, add it to your list and forge ahead.

Fashion Your Figure was a generalized movement program based on prevalent problems of many, many women. This book will take a close look and a more intensive approach, though the underlying philosophy of exercise as a necessary but pleasant and regular part of life certainly applies.

You will use the program as you wish, but we'd like to suggest a method that we think will best help you integrate it into your daily schedule and then permanently into your life. It will change as you need it to change. You should modify it for special situations and crises.

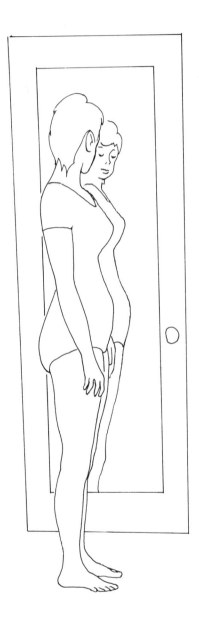

First, you have to close the gap between what you are, physically, and what you think you are. We look at ourselves with wishful eyes, so with the best intention in the world, it is easy to cheat. Don't do it. Take some comfort in the fact that most women look better with their clothes on than off.

To find out where to start, strip and stand in front of a big mirror (a hand mirror constitutes cheating). If you can't bear it, put on leotards or tights which will lessen the shock but won't obscure the problem.

Now take a pen and note pad and, starting at your head, take merciless inventory. Where does your head sit on your neck? Is your chin way out? Do your shoulders go forward more easily than down (and have you had trouble fitting into blouses lately?)? Is there a lump at the back of your neck?

Go down the body listing all the questionable spots in one column. Now close your eyes and start over. With the same surgical eye, see in your mind the area you are thinking of and how you would like it to look. Be realistic. If you have wide, wide pelvic bones, you'll never achieve whippy hips. Where do you want your neck to sit? How much flab will come off those thighs, in terms of your overall body build? Don't fantasize and don't dream.

Take it exactly from where you are and you may

be surprised to find how much of it is all right. Maybe you have a magnificent head carriage but are a blob from shoulder to knee. Perhaps the whole torso is gorgeous, but the arms lag and the thighs sag. Get a clear picture of what you have to correct.

Now find out what you want to preserve. In the second column, list your assets. You want exercise that will help you keep your good points on the credit side of your ledger. You can call it preventive exercise, or movement to keep something from happening.

As you read the book, mark or note which exercises you feel will work for your specific problems. There are several for each. You can use all of them or pick the one or ones that you like to do. Bear in mind how much time you want to spend, what you want to get done, and then put together a program for yourself.

At first, we strongly advise that you do this program at a given time and place every day. Normally we look on a rigid program as a type of stopgap; but if you consider it as a kind of emergency necessity until you get used to it, the routine will prepare you sooner for incorporating it into your life on a more relaxed schedule.

Try your first program for two weeks. By this time you should be well enough along, if you have been faithful, to take Sundays off. Go back to the book and look at the exercises again. Substitute

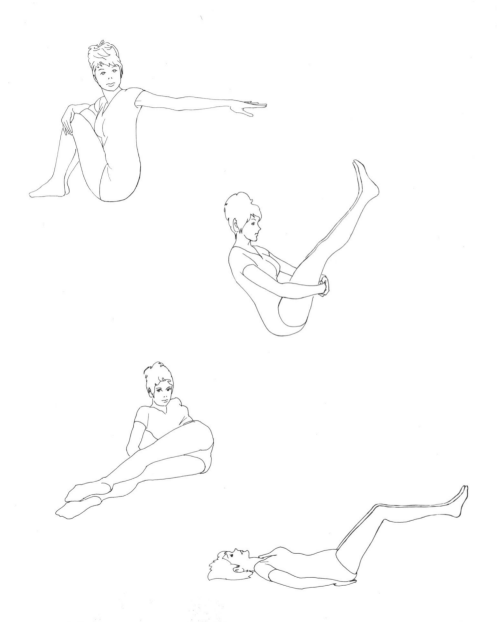

if you wish. You will be well aware, by then, that they overlap — just as muscles overlap particular body areas — and that some of them (as in the chapters on posture, waist and abdomen, hips and thighs, and in the final chapter on tension) are excellent overall movements. Reshuffle them but, as you experiment with them, make yourself a note file about what each exercise (after a fair trial) does for you, even if it is no more than to say "Hard" or "Easy" or "Fun." In your own program, alternate the hard ones and the easy ones.

At the end of a month, you should be perfectly confident about what you are doing. There should be a perceptible change in the firmness and suppleness of your body. And you will want to add some of the exercises to the things you do either outside your own home, or outside your exercise routine. To this end, we have added a paragraph or more to each chapter (or at the end of a specific section) about what we call The Throwaways — brief movements you can do when you are sitting at a desk, or taking a coffee break, or even watching television. Work them in, but not frivolously or with an attitude of "Isn't this silly?" — because it isn't. You should do them as you would take a prescribed medicine, but you prescribe the time.

At the end of two months, you should drop the whole thing for a couple of days, stand off, and look at it. Is it helping as you want it to? If not, why not? If so, are you ready to cut back on some parts of it? The idea is to get a program flexible enough to serve you with the same kind of variety that your own life has. Keep a reference file of what works best. Make a special program from it for particular events. Plan how to use exercise before the baby and, even more importantly, after the baby comes. How about a special three-week schedule to get ready for summer? A modified crash for after those caloric holidays?

The important step is to have tailored a program that fits your needs as you see them. It will be your basic activity schedule, though it will change when you need it to change. Once you have your body in hand, and know how it responds to exercise and to this kind of rhythmed order, you can be ready for what comes.

In any case, you are on your own. That is the severest discipline of all.

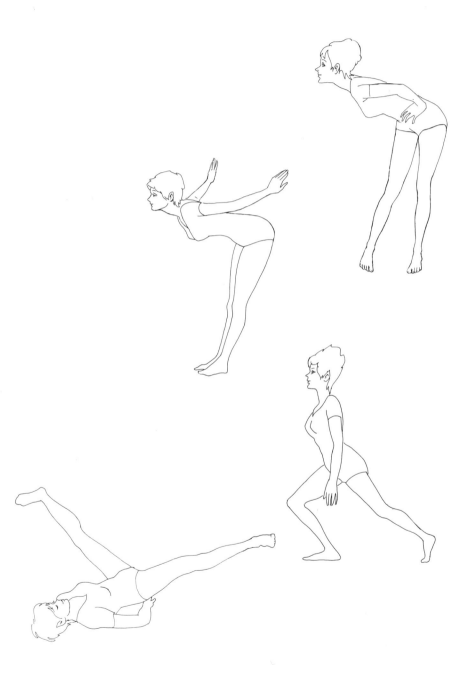

CHAPTER 3

POSTURE AND CARRIAGE—
FRONT AND BACK

Posture is body sculpture.

It is subliminal shorthand to say how you feel about yourself. Notice the way you carry your body when you are on top of everything. Notice the difference when some of the well-being has drained away.

Of course, you could have a weak back, but if you did, you'd know it by now and that would be a different ball game. The best idea, if all signals are normal, is to check your self-esteem gauge and have a look at the laziness level. It is the latter that results in chronic slouch and slump.

You know how to stand in good posture, how to fold over and roll your spine back to get everything aligned. The tuck is the key. When your buttock muscles are pressed together, the pelvic bones have nowhere to go except where they belong. That straightens the whole line, all the way up and down.

This does not mean you are going to be straight, tidy, and plumb all the time — that would be self-conscious and dreary. But note, as you do stand in good posture, that this is the proper association your bones, muscles, and organs should have with each other. Try to maintain the relativity, whether you are standing, sitting, lying, or learning.

To know how it all ought to feel, stand with legs apart, knees loose, then round the back, and hang over dangling your arms in front. Curl the spine up slowly, keeping the pelvis tucked (if you

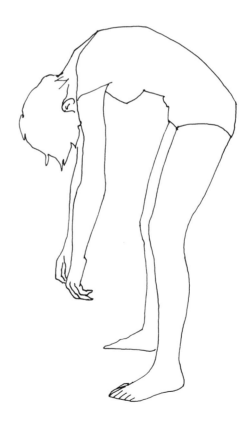

13

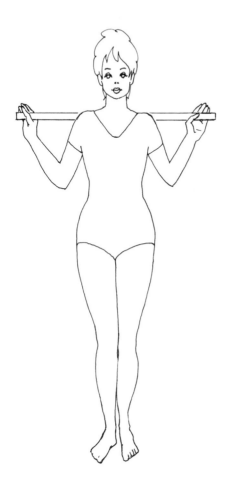

squeeze the buttocks together, it has to stay that way), and come up to a standing position with your body on a loose plumb line.

If you keep this general body position, sitting and standing, you can evade the round shoulders and widow's hump that are the diplomas of tension and sloppy body position.

The hump is caused by leading with the chin, which may reflect either aggression or defense on your part but is a bad position for either battle. It can get worse as you get older and forget how much more comfortable the correct position is.

When you are standing as you should, a pole or yardstick, held lightly in the hands, will rest comfortably and flatly across the upper back without any squeezing of the shoulder blades. Continuous attention to the posture of your shoulders can prevent or minimize (as your case may be) that dinner roll just back of the armpits.

Tight, front-thrust shoulders pull those back muscles up and forward for so long that when you finally get the shoulders where they belong the pulled tissues sag. This kind of bad posture is also part of the reason for the other roll — that one across the top of the bra in the back.

Correcting bad habits, especially posture ones, is hard. When you have let the back slump too long, it is going to tell you with pain that it wishes to be let alone. Once you understand the proper relation of the pelvic tuck and the lifted rib cage, many back problems become simply a matter of faithful drill. You will have to undergo some discomfort at first; after all, you created the crisis yourself, and so you must schedule a daily therapeutic routine until those knots begin to untie. Then you can incorporate your drill into a wider general program.

Babies often create back problems that didn't have to happen. New mothers often don't realize the extreme importance of an immediate exercise program after the birth; because they don't know how to stand, they carry their new burdens wrong. The posture exercises, and those in the chapter on waist and abdomen, are especially suited for post-natal work. You will want to clear them with your own doctor, of course, but at no other time in your life will fitness be more important than in the years when your children are young — for your sake and theirs. So start to exercise before they come, and keep it up as they grow.

The following exercises put some emphasis on the spine and back, but are excellent for overall posture control.

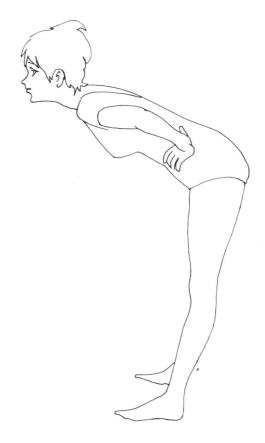

1. Stand with feet apart, turned slightly out, hands on hips. Bend forward, back straight and eyes ahead, coming as far toward a 90-degree angle as is comfortable. Accommodate the strain with a slight bend in the knees, if necessary. Curl the spine under, beginning at the base, and roll

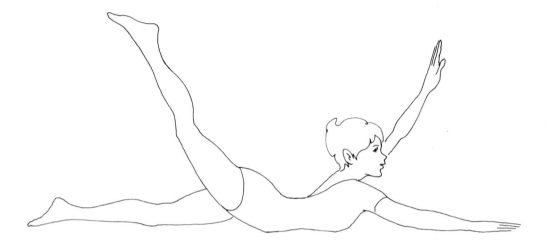

back up to standing position. The curl will start when you tuck the pelvis, so let your stomach help. Keep the shoulders in line. They will want to bunch. Don't let them. Eight times.

Graduate Variation: Same exercise, but as you bend forward, extend your arms in front, bringing them down as you start the spinal curl and letting them go back to the hips.

2. Lie on the floor on your stomach, chin on the floor, arms stretched out in front with palms down on the floor. Raise the right arm and the left leg at the same time, letting your head come up with your arm. Hold for five counts and slowly lower them. Reverse the sides: left arm with right leg. Four times.

This exercise strengthens the muscles of the middle back and is helpful in easing tension there.

Graduate Variation: Raise both arms and count five, then lower. Raise both legs and count five, then lower.

Doctorate Degree: Raise everything at once, leaving nothing much on the floor but your stomach. Count five and take a rest.

3. Stand with feet apart, arms lifted overhead but relaxed, shoulders down. Swing the arms down to the side and, in the same rhythmic swish, fold the body down, letting the head droop, bending the knees, and relaxing the back. On the next beat, swing the arms back up and let the momentum pull the body back up to standing position. This is one long continuous movement and you stop only at the beginning and end.

4. Sit on the floor in a cross-legged position with your back pressed against the wall all the way up from the base to the back of the head — or as much of it as you can manage. Breathe in deeply, raising your arms with elbows relaxed, and put as much of your arms as you can against the wall, without letting loose with your back or raising your shoulders. Your arms will now be in a gentle U-shape above your head. It is harder than it looks because everything wants to come down and out. Don't let it, for a slow four counts, then relax and breathe out, and in another four counts collapse down in a heap in front of your ankles.

Work up to eight times. This attacks the baggy tissues both in front and in back of your armpits, smoothes and firms the upper back, and gets your shoulders accustomed to staying where they ought.

The Throwaways

For good habits out of bad habits: slump where you sit, being sure the tailbone is against the back of a chair or solid surface. Curl the body back against the chair, lifting the torso, which should pull in the abdomen.

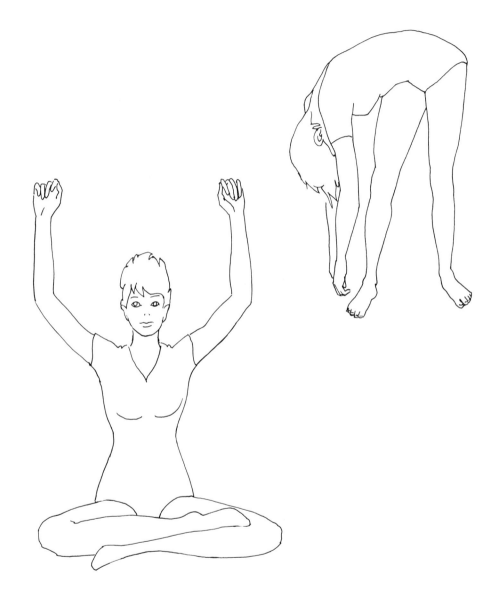

17

Swing your arms when you walk. Somewhere along the way, this got to be considered showy, but it is excellent exercise, especially in the posture context.

Look straight ahead, or at least keep your eyes ahead, when you walk; but keep your chin in re-

CHAPTER 4

FACE, HEAD, AND NECK—
THE COMMAND POST

serve. We've said it before, but it is important to remember that if you lead with your chin, you throw your whole body out of line.

If you stay in good standing, the dividends are in your looks.

The best thing you can do for your face is to have happy thoughts behind it.

If the body is the mirror of the feelings, then the face is their magnifying glass. What you do and don't do are faithfully reflected — sometimes unfortunately, as in the case of too much sun, too little sleep, too much tension, too much rich food, improper cleansing, inadequate lubrication. Facial happiness comes with the obverse of the above, plus a witty and reasoned acceptance of things as they are.

Cosmetic surgery (once called "plastic" and used only in major emergencies) has made giant strides in the last few years. If there is a compelling professional or emotional reason for you to resort to it, the safety factor is high and the techniques are magnificent. It is, nevertheless, a form of artifice, and the artificial image invariably runs into problems of maintenance.

Therefore, if you can manage it, accept your face, with its inevitable lines, as the diary of a varied journey. That is the most comfortable and, in the end, the most beautiful solution.

What exercise does for the face is to improve the circulation and strengthen the muscle tone. These are very important factors at any age, beginning with the very young, but they are accessories; the final beauty of the face must come from behind it.

In fact, don't be drastic with any facial exercise. The simple fact of communication gives your face a great deal of exercise. What you want to hit with a planned program is the relaxation of muscles already — and normally — heavily used. There is no need to deepen the landmarks.

1. Begin in bed (O happy day!), lying on your back, arms resting back above your head, and knees raised in a tent. (You can tuck while you are resting.) Open your mouth and drop your jaw as far as possible. This is what you do when you yawn, so you probably will. Close the mouth slowly. Eight times.

This very simple exercise helps tighten the chin and firm the laugh lines that put your mouth in parentheses.

2. Sitting with knees apart, drop your head between them and shake it liberally, like a wet dog. Four times.

3. *To relax the eye muscles:* Sit on a chair, hands in lap, back relaxed but straight. Close your eyes, tilt your head back as far as is comfortable, and open the eyes wide. Bring head forward onto your chest, closing your eyes as you come.

4. Sitting or lying, close your eyes and look up, down, and to each side. Then make the entire circle, as if you were scanning the perimeter of your sight, with your eyes shut. Four times.

5. *For those chin muscles:* Open your mouth slightly and jut your lower jaw forward in front of the upper jaw, then return it to its natural alignment. Don't be drastic. Four times.

The Throwaway

The Fish Bowl: Sit, knees crossed. Pucker the lips as far forward as possible (kissing gourami). Pull back into a tight smile (fighting betta). Relax with a session of flapping the lower lip against the upper one, carrying the whole lower jaw (beached guppy). Four times.

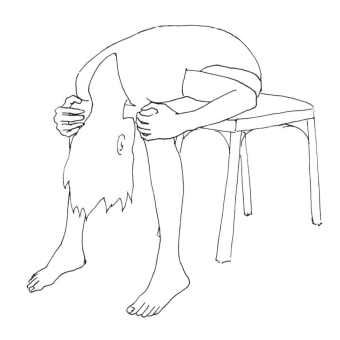

THE HEAD AND NECK

There is an old saying about putting your best foot forward when you wish to appear to advantage. Unfortunately, what is usually farthest forward in any such situation is your head. Very often your chin is thrust out in front of that.

This does not necessarily imply aggressiveness. It may be a position of attention, of absorption and involvement, of sympathy. But, whatever the nature of the attitudes that produce it, the result is the same. The body goes out of plumb, off balance, and the muscles strain to do what the bones ought to be doing to get it back. Where do you hurt when you have been under any kind of stress? At the back of your neck, of course.

The head should sit directly on the spine, as if you were suspended by the tips of your ears. If you tuck your pelvis properly and keep that head in alignment, the rest of your body comes naturally into good posture. Your head is relaxed, flexible, responsive. Your neck becomes more than just a hinge; it is a beautiful control channel between the command center, which is the head, and the action operation, which is the rest of you.

One word of warning about any exercises that involve your neck and head. Do nothing abruptly! Do not strain! The neck is the last stretch before a whole complex of important nerves reach the protection of the bony skull. They are vulnerable. Handle them with care.

1. *To do penance for past sins:* Stand in good posture and let your body slump forward with the head leading until it hangs over your chest. Your arms are loose in front of your knees. Now shake out, both arms and head, lolling from side to side, eyes closed. Breathe in deeply, raise your head slowly, and come out to erect posture. Six times.

2. Tailor-sit against the wall, back straight, shoulders to the flat surface but not tense, back of head against the wall. Now relax the chin down to the chest, feeling the pull of those muscles that bunch into the neck. Try to roll back up the wall so that all of the back of your neck is touching it. This is impossible, of course, but it is the feeling you wish to achieve. What you do is bring your head back to starting position. It works not only on the back muscles but on the saggy ones in front. Six times.

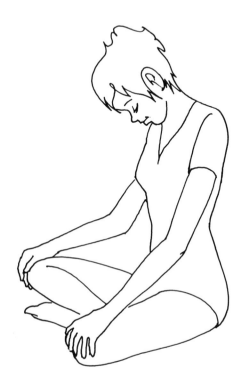

3. *For overrelaxed chin muscles:* Lift your chin as if searching for something in the sky. Your shoulders and upper body will lift slightly. Open your mouth and drop the jaw, then lower the head to close the mouth. Let the lift out of the shoulders at the same time. Eight times.

The Throwaway

Sitting or standing, look straight ahead and tilt your head slowly to the right as if to rest it on your shoulder (not too far and don't strain). Then roll

23

the head forward over the chest into the same tilted position on the other shoulder. Straighten slowly to the look-ahead position. Repeat in the opposite direction. Eight times slowly.

CHAPTER 5

SHOULDERS, ARMS, AND HANDS — THE DOERS

It is somehow a good idea to do all these neck exercises with closed eyes. It seems to promote relaxation and helps you concentrate on performing steadily but gently.

You can't go back, and your shoulders, especially, shouldn't try!

There is no way to gauge the harm that has been done by that ancient admonition, from parent to child down the generations: "Hold your shoulders back." All the wrong things happen when you do: the spine curves into a sway, the pelvis is pushed out of line, and the hips go out. Only the fingernails are unaffected, but the resultant strain will probably get you into the stage where you will bite *them*.

When this phrase comes to mind, edit it promptly to "Lift your chest and let your shoulders hang out," which is to say, press those shoulders down and out. Don't even think "back."

1. Stand in good posture against a wall, then move free of it, keeping shoulders down and out. Raise elbows to the shoulder height and touch your

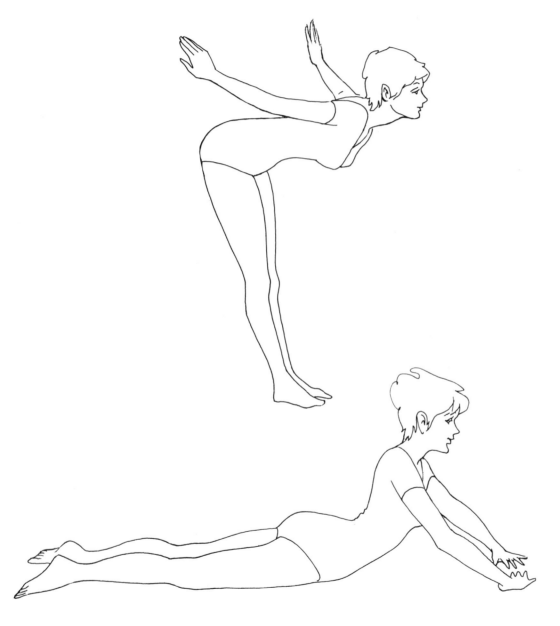

finger tips in front of you, keeping chin and eyes straight ahead. Open arms forward, out and back (as if you were going into a swan dive) and, breaking at the waist, let the upper body lean forward in one piece to balance the arm position. You should accomplish this on a count of four, breathing in. On another count of four, breathe out and return to your first position. Eight times.

This puts emphasis on the lower part of the arm-pit, including that troublesome pile above the breast area.

2. Lie flat on your stomach, feet relaxed and toes out. Bend your arms, fingers touching at the tips, and rest your forehead on them. Press up, lifting your chest from the floor. The weight will go first to your forearms, then to the flattened palms of your hands, as you come up as far as is comfortable. Your spine will be swayed but the stretch will be across the front of your shoulders and your upper chest. Count four up, breathing in, and four down, breathing out. Work up to eight times.

There are bonuses all over in this one — neck, waist, and lower abdomen. It is a magnificent exercise!

The Throwaway

Circle right shoulder eight times, bringing it forward, up, down, and back. Same motion with left shoulder. Then do both at once.

THE ARMS

The arms suggest what the hands say.

People speak often of beautiful and expressive hands, more seldom of beautiful and expressive arms. They are considered a working arrangement between the body and the hands. Only in special contexts do we isolate them — in the dance, of course, and in novels written about the nostalgic charms of feminine limbs in soft fabric by summer twilight.

It is too bad. Arms have their own carriage, an almost separate posture. The outer arm held just out from the shoulder with a slightly rounded wrist and inturned hand is one of the most beautiful of the body's lines. The inner arm, in the same position, is one of the most sensual. This is one of the most intimate of the public parts of the body and should never be underestimated or neglected. This is as true for men as for women.

All our lives we use the arm below the elbow relatively correctly, but we get lazy with the upper arm and it turns into a safe deposit for spare tissue. A fat bank. Even with golf.

1. Sitting tailor position, or standing in good posture (you should watch the pelvic tuck: arm exercises tend to lead the tuck astray into a sway), raise arms overhead, palms out and backs touching. Bend elbows and press arms out to the sides,

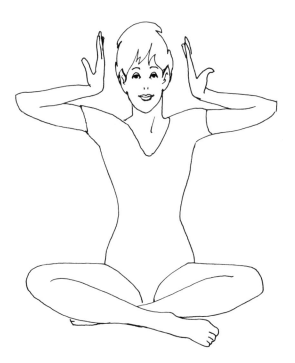

stretching through finger tips. Come back overhead. Breathe in as arms go up, out as they come down. Eight times.

2. Sitting or standing, arms out to the sides, palms up. Turn palms back and make a fist and grip tightly for four slow counts. Relax, let elbows bend down, and drop arms to the side. Breathe in for grip, out as you drop. Eight times.

The two exercises noted in Chapter 11 for use with weights are excellent arm exercises and may be used in this grouping, without the weights.

The Throwaway

Hold your body in good posture, relaxed and with the arms out, and shake both arms from the shoulders through loose finger tips, as if you were a tree trying to free itself of leaves. Count four for each set of shakes.

THE HANDS

None of this is to belittle the human hand, which is certainly a masterpiece of beauty, planning, and utility. Hands are the outermost extensions of ourselves. They tell more about us than we would perhaps like to have known.

For a long time the hand was a cosmetic extravagance, and for some it still is. In the crackling action of today's society, the well-groomed, understated hand is smarter. Men are paying more attention to their hands. Women are being more subtle about theirs — shorter nails, paler polish shades, but always such good elemental care as cream for the skin, oil for cuticles, and those dry side sections that are so seductive to the nail-biter or -nipper, and no polish at all if you can't keep it from chipping. There are lots of drastic things to do for special occasions — extravagant paste-ons, beauty patches, rings, and bangles, but these are usually one-night stands. We are talking about the hands with which you cook dinner, serve tennis balls, type, and garden.

It is the use of your hand which makes it beautiful, whatever its anatomical structure. Short, stubby fingers can be marvelously expressive. The most exquisite, fairy-tale slender, meticulously manicured hand is dull if it says nothing about you.

Keep the hands clean, groomed, and agile. A good way to start is to fall back on the piano students' standby, Mr. Hanon and his finger exercises — his first one, in fact. You won't need a piano. The fact that the book is called *The Virtuoso Pianist* might even encourage you.

1. *Mr. Hanon's First Exercise:* Rest your arm and wrist on a table, the hand easily arched, the thumb resting alongside, the finger tips on the table. Now, striking with the thumb first, go up the scale one finger at a time, and back down. This is a relaxed version of what you do when you are important or angry. Ten times with each hand, and *not* angrily.

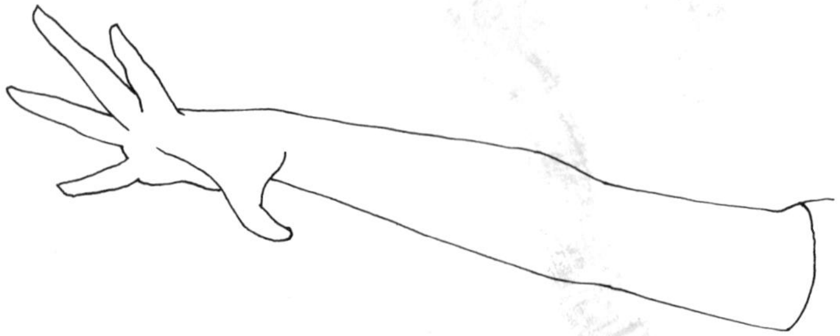

2. With the elbows held in to the body, life your hands as if you were a rabbit with loose fingers. Circle the hands from the wrist, four times in, four times out. This is good for firming the lower arm muscles as well as relaxing the entire hand.

The Throwaway

Make a fist, relaxed but still a fist, then scatter the fingers outward in a calculated stretch. In and out four times.

These exercises are good no matter how young you are, but they are invaluable as you grow older,

CHAPTER 6

BREASTS, DIAPHRAGM, AND UPPER

BACK — THE HIGH MIDDLE

especially when arthritic conditions attack one finger or another. In such cases, exercise is vital — not strenuous or continuous, but planned and regular.

Jean Stafford once wrote an exquisite short story about a beautiful woman who destroyed herself when she found that there was no way to disguise the aging hand.

And there is none. Your hands will age, for some people faster and in different ways than for others. Marks will come in the skin, and some knuckles will gnarl. Accept this equitably. Do not try to hide your hands. Do not be self-conscious about them. They are rewards for a busy life. They are what you have done.

As you lift out of a casual slouch, or haul yourself from a television slump to a good sitting position, you can take some note of the magical things that happen because those muscles on which a lot of the upper half of your body hangs have been given help from back and below.

The little molding just above the waist disappears, the tension goes out of the upper back, and the breasts come proudly forward. The diaphragm and upper back are good places to do preventive exercises, since they are awfully hard to get to once the fat tissue has found them and made a home.

The bosom, more than any other single physical characteristic, represents the essence of womanliness. Its fashion changes, but its style is eternal. No matter what the status of its owner, the bosom is her. Some years it is flat; some seasons button-bosoms are high style. For a long time the breasts went, by one means or another, up and out to a point. At the moment the look is inclined to be comfortable and relatively unconfined. But at any time, they remain the distinguishing symbol of woman's part in the human picture — a source of sexual pleasure, of nourishment for her young, an outer mark of her inner mystique.

The size of your breasts depends upon the way you are built and is as genetic in origin as the shape of your face or the length of your legs. Their size also depends on the amount of weight you carry, for the breast is made up of spongy tissue and fat. The only muscles involved are the little patch around the nipple and the all-important pectorals from which this tissue is slung in a masterly cross-web from above, below, and across.

You can get rid of the fat. The spongy tissue will sag, inevitably, with age, and the only thing you can do about that is surgery. Tremendous strides have been made in this field, and thousands of women now take advantage of it in safety. But there is a great deal you yourself can do about your breasts if you take care of the pectorals — those vital carrying muscles. The loose, braless look is only for the young and firm, but even youth is not relieved from the obligation of maintenance.

You presumably don't need to be told about breast health. If you have not already, do please learn from your doctor how to do your own lump-detecting. If you feel anything in there that shouldn't be, get right to him and see about it. Breast cancer is common, but it is nowhere near the specter it was before women learned to be forewarned and act quickly.

If you slump, the undue and unnecessary weight will make those shoulder muscles stretch. It is easier to prevent the lag than it is to get rid of it. The slump denies the breasts the support of the crucial side muscles and the cunning crosstension inserted into them.

So to work with the muscles that you can get at.

1. *For the breasts:* Sit with feet apart and in good posture, pelvis tucked. Bring your elbows up and clench fists into the bosom. Maintaining the fists, spread your arms forward, out to the side, and slightly back, bending the upper body forward a little. Now bounce the arms backward slightly for ten counts. (Keep the pelvis tucked and don't let your lower back go into a sway. This provides the

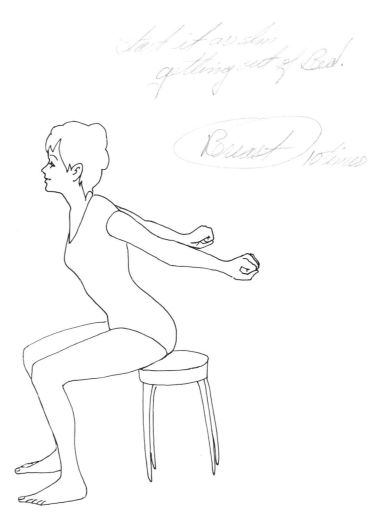

33

side bonus of tummy tightening.) Come back to first position. Eight times.

This exercise is also good for the forward armpit area and the spread just above it.

2. *For the diaphragm and rib cage:* Standing, clench right hand into a fist at the side. Bend arm at elbow and, keeping tension, raise the fist forward, up into the shoulder and on up directly overhead, straight armed. Bring it back to shoulder position and down to side, then relax. Repeat with left arm; then with both arms at once. Do the entire exercise eight times. (For added pull, use a three-pound weight or an empty soft-drink bottle in each hand.) This exercise will come as close as anything to reaching the muscles underneath the breasts.

3. *For the breasts:* Sit on the floor, back straight, and hug knees to chest with your right hand on the left knee and vice versa. Breathing in, open right arm to the side, out and back, turning your upper body to follow but keeping the back straight. Make the sweep from front to back to front again in one continuous motion, feeling it in the side breast area and the back muscles above the bra line. Repeat with the left arm. Entire exercise eight times.

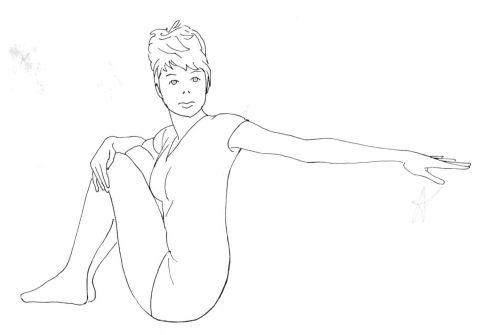

4. *For the diaphragm:* Lie on your stomach, chin on the floor, hands clasped over the buttocks, palms up. Keeping your pelvis tucked to relieve back strain, breathe in and push palms toward feet, pulling shoulders and upper body off floor. It does not matter how high or low you go, but you must feel the pull across the top of the breasts. Breathe out and relax. Eight times.

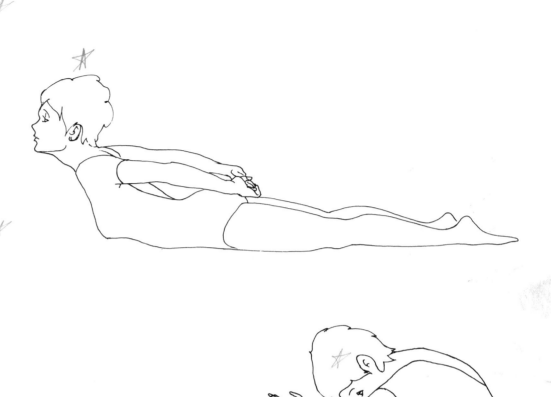

5. *For the upper back:* Sit on the floor, legs out in front, knees loose, back straight, and arms loose to sides. Breathe in and scoop the arms forward, breaking at the waist, over the knees and up in front, as if you were trying to trap an armful of air. When arms are overhead, open them wide to the sides and breathe out as the back straightens. Drop to the first position. Eight times.

The Throwaway

Sitting straight and with elbows raised out to the sides, jam the hands together at the joint between thumb and forefinger. It doesn't have to be a collision, but the meeting should be strong enough so you can see the muscles leap across your upper breast area and feel the pull across the back. Eight times.

CHAPTER 7

WAIST AND ABDOMEN
— THE LOW MIDDLE

We will define the waist as the area between the bottom of the rib cage and the top of the hips, and you will be wise to note that it is usually the first to go.

For our purposes, we will define the abdomen as the fleshy area in front of the waist and below it, before the legs branch from the trunk. The waist is easier to deal with since, by its swivel nature, it gets more exercise in the course of everyday activity. The abdomen and the all-important stomach muscles get only what exercise we give them consciously.

When we are younger, the tissues are firm and more resilient, as we are ourselves. We twist and turn more, move more, and are more relaxed, so that the stress-and-release pattern that helps us keep firm does its work naturally.

When we are older, more tissue collects there. It gets less resilient at about the same rate we do. The bad sitting and standing habits that were relatively harmless in our salad years (because we didn't stay still very long anyway) become deadly. The tissue settles around into a permanent girdle.

Some of this is to be expected: very few women stay exactly the same size. But there is little reason not to keep the same firmness.

Housework used to help. Back in the days when there was a washboard, a clothesline, even a washing machine with a hand wringer, what you did for your family had a healthy physicality. It also made

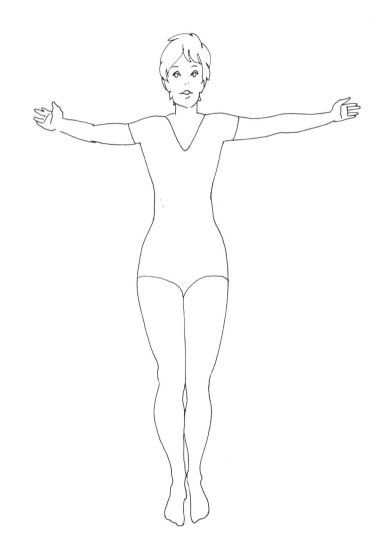

you tired, and modern technology does not like ladies to be tired. So now there are all kinds of wonderful machines that do your work for you.

Since nobody is going to opt a return to the washboard, what to do?

The first thing is to think UP. Just the mental impetus to lift your body starts an impulse in the right direction. Go up before you go over (into a car), out (of a chair), or down (into bed).

1. *Rope Pulling* (to lift the stuff out of the waist): Stand straight, legs apart, and reach up overhead, one arm at a time, with the weight on the opposite leg. Pull up as if you were lifting your body by hauling it up two parallel ropes. Keep the face to the front. Sixteen times.

Variation: Change ropes. Reach for the left-hand rope with the right arm and vice versa. This intensifies the stretch. Sixteen times.

2. Standing with feet apart, pelvis tucked, and hands on hips, keep face to front and without moving feet bend the body as far to the right as is comfortable. Then bring it up and over to the left, feeling the pull in the side waist muscles. Eight times.

Variation: Bend body to the right, as above, then twist the upper body to face the right, and bend forward over the right leg, chin up. Turn upper body back to the tilt position and bring it up erect. The pelvis will come untucked and the

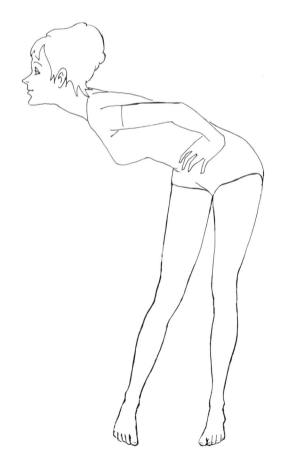

knees loosen to accommodate the pull in the back, but both should return to their first position as the body moves upward. Same to the left. Eight times.

3. *The Oval Vegetable Dish:* Sit on the floor, back straight, feet flat, and knees raised with the arms in a loose loop in front. The arms keep position, circling with the body, through the entire exercise. Describe an oval with the upper body, arms leading with hips as pivot; that is, circle to the right over the hip, then back, tucking under the hips, then left, and around to the first position. Reverse.

As muscles gain strength, you can make your oval wider and closer to the floor. When you really want to work at it, use a three-pound weight or dumbbell in your hands. Be sure you tuck under the hips as you go back. This is what puts the pull in the waist. If you feel it in your back, your position is faulty.

4. *For the abdomen:* Lie flat on your back and bend your knees up, breathing in until your legs are at a 90-degree angle with your body. Pulling in the stomach muscles, propel your knees forward — as if to push your feet against an imaginary wall — as far as you can go without moving the abdomen muscles or letting the spine leave the floor. The legs from knees down stay always roughly parallel to the floor. When it hurts, pull back, breathing out. Eight times.

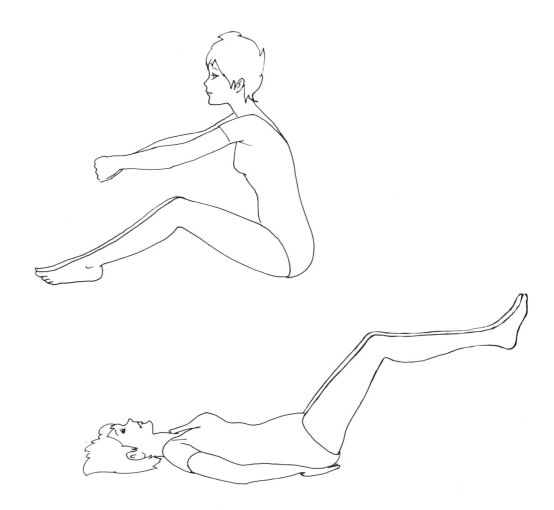

5. *For the abdomen:* Lie flat on your back and bend knees up over stomach. Straighten your right leg and begin to lower it, heel leading, keeping the spine on the floor and the stomach muscles taut. In a slow scissor, straighten the left leg and lower it as the right one comes up. Neither ever touches the floor or goes down far enough to make the back hurt. You may put your hands under the lower buttocks if that makes things easier. Eight times.

CHAPTER 8

HIPS AND THIGHS—
THE FAT BANK

The Throwaway

Every chance you get, squeeze your buttocks together and pull your stomach muscles in. This pressure action affects muscles all the way up to the waist and is an invaluable strengthener.

It is your bonus that most exercises which are designed primarily for hips and thighs are also major helps for undisciplined stomachs and waist bands. Bear it in mind.

When four-footed animal became two-footed animal, he lost half his immediate support from the earth. Upright man must use his pelvis as a kind of fulcrum to help distribute his weight and to preserve his body balance.

For a woman, the pelvic area is even more important, for it is the frame within which she carries on her vital procreative activities; her support during the period she is carrying her child. It is also a reservoir for tissue. Youthful action, childbearing and child care, the busy life of the early years usually burn that tissue up. But as the activities slow down, the reservoir is not emptied so easily. As a bald fact, it is fat's favorite resting place. It is certainly the most difficult area from which to clear excess weight.

In our observation, through years of teaching both exercise and dance, the carriage of the upper body has a great effect on the development of the lower body. The hip area, unlikely as it may seem, is the body's attic, the repository of all the tissue that can't be put to use somewhere else. The accumulation doesn't have to happen, but many things make it predictable. We sit too much. We eat too much. Then, because, quite naturally, we wish to look our best, we counteract our laziness with artificial means. We wear girdles that are tight, even stayed. This makes us flat where it shows, in the waist and stomach, but what is left has to go somewhere, and the nearest haven is the inner thigh, which finally gets flabby, and the outer hip, which develops a chronic bulge. It is hard to get rid of this weight, and so it is much better if you can manage to evade both deposits.

The best way to begin is to practice carrying your entire body properly so consistently that you finally do it all the time. Most people get the idea of the Tuck easily — it is that slight underthrust of the pelvic bones that aligns the body, supporting the upper part and distributing equitably what the hips and legs will carry. The Lift, which should accompany the Tuck, is somehow not so easy to understand. Think of a cord coming out of the top of your head and holding you erect. You know somehow that it will pull your rib cage up (as it goes up a little when you lift), settle your shoulders down, and that it will be gentle and comfortable. At the same time, if done correctly, it will pull a lot of that stuff up out of the hip area before it takes permanent residence. When sitting, you should think of yourself not as resting on a block, but as hanging on a hook. It is comfortable if you do it right.

The first thing to do about it is to walk more — more and longer and more briskly. This is the best exercise for the whole complex — bones and tissue alike. You cannot start a steady walking program too early, and if you are wise you will never abandon it.

1. To get in the mood indoors, you might try the silent rock. Sit on the floor, back erect, feet straight in front, and rock stiffly from side to side, balancing with a hand here and there if necessary. Sixteen times.

2. To deal with what you have already accumulated on the hips, try a high bicycle. The standard bicycle exercise, as you know, is to lie on your back, raise your legs and pedal in the air. The high bicycle carries your body up to where the weight rests on your upper back and shoulders, supported by your hands on your hips. Your feet should be straight up in the air as you start to pedal. Work up a reasonable speed. Pedal twenty-four times.

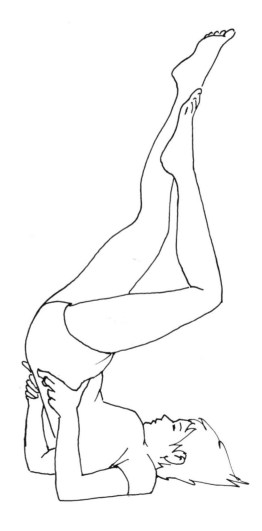

Rest, then do twenty-four more. This gets to muscles that little else will reach.

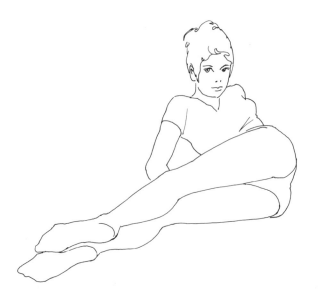

3. To deal with those disgusting little buns that just fit your palms when you rest your hands in back right below the waist, lie on your back and raise your upper body to rest on the elbows. Bend the legs into the chest, then roll to the right and straighten the legs. Circle them up and over to the left (still straight), bending again only as you bring them back to center. Reverse. You will know you are in proper position if you hit the pones each time your straight legs move across. Eight times.

4. Lie on the right side all the way down. Lift your head and support it with your right hand and elbow. Put the other hand palm down on the floor in front to keep you balanced on the point of one hip. Bend the top leg forward and in, keeping it always parallel to the floor, then stretch it down and back, heel leading, slightly behind the bottom leg. Repeat the forward-back action sixteen times, progressively faster. Roll over and do it on the other side, sixteen times.

Variation: Lying in the same position, keep the top leg straight and raise it enough to describe a stiff-kneed circle in the air, sixteen times each side, working up to thirty-two.

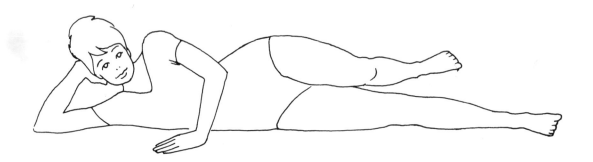

5. *To attack the outer thigh hillock:* Lie on the floor on your back. Pull up, letting your elbows support your upper body. Draw your knees up to your chest. Keeping your knees drawn up and leaving your upper body in the same position, roll your lower body as far as possible to the right over the hip — up, out, and back around to the chest. Repeat to the other side. You will be describing a horizontal figure eight with the crossover where your knees come to your chest on each roll. Do this sixteen times, breathing in as you roll over, out as you start back for the chest each time.

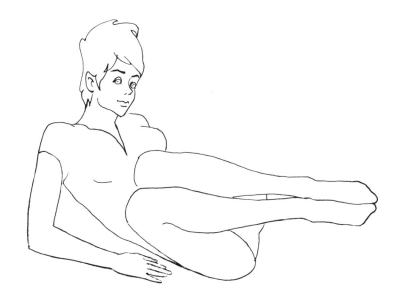

THE THIGHS

1. Put your weight on the left leg and let the right one come forward with a little weight on the ball of the foot or on the toe. Then bend the left leg down as far as you can comfortably, echoing the bend in the other leg. Don't let the hips loose; they go down too! Sixteen times each leg.

Graduate Variation: Lift the right leg off the floor as you do your bends. Not high, but enough to get more weight into the upper thigh.

2. Stand on your right leg. Raise the left leg, knee bent, to waist level, lower it again, and without pause turn it out to the side (as near to a right angle to the first position as possible). Raise and lower again. There should be no pause between lifts; the leg should go like a pendulum, up and down and side and down. Sixteen times for each

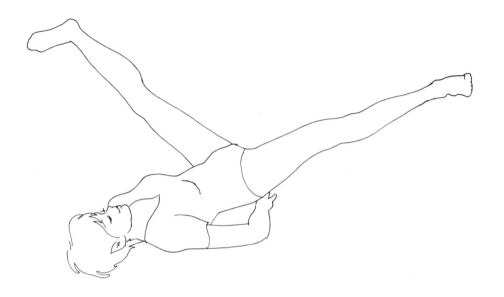

leg. If you are young and very frisky, raise the knee as high as you can, but the work gets done satisfactorily if you go only as high as the knee.

3. Lie on your side, head supported by elbow and hand, your stomach muscles firmly in, and your pelvic area tucked. Lift the top leg, foot flexed, and heel leading, and make a series of small circles, breathing in for two and out for two. Sixteen times on each side.

4. Lie on your back, hands under your buttocks. Breathe in, tighten your stomach muscles, and raise your legs straight up, feet flexed and heels leading. Now let the legs go into a split, as far as

CHAPTER 9

KNEES, LEGS, ANKLES, AND
FEET—RAPID TRANSIT

is comfortable, toes facing in, and bounce gently seven times. Bring them in and relax on the count of eight. Repeat.

The Throwaways

Standing in good posture, swing each leg backward and forward sixteen times. You may want to hold on to a chair at first. It is an exercise in balance when you have mastered it.

Another excellent hip and thigh exercise is the simple knee bend, or what the dancers call a *plié*. Stand with your feet apart and make as if to sit, then come back up. Breathing deeply in and out, needless to say.

Nature has a way of working her own balance system with our physical endowments. In such areas as the hips and thighs, she gives us great bones and lets us hang on them what we will, usually too much.

With some of the other equipment, you take what you get. Legs and knees come in that basket.

A knee, for instance, is a knee — the body's workhorse. Often it is asked to appear better than it can be made to look. The nicest thing you can do for it is not to mistreat it, and to keep it flexible.

1. *For the knees:* Sit on the floor, or in a straight chair. Clasp your hands together just under the knees and bring your legs up to your chest in a loose hug. Now make a V-shape of yourself, straightening the legs and stretching them up as far as possible. If you creak, you'll know it was time to oil the hinges. Lower the legs. Eight times.

The conformation of your legs is another birthright that you must take and live with. If you have big calves, keep them beautifully groomed, nourished with whatever cream you fancy, and give them sun in the summer — not too much: that mahogany look is not nearly so exciting now that we know more about the relation of overexposure to skin cancer. Otherwise, think of those legs as if you had borrowed them from Alexandra Danilova.

There are not many corrective exercises for big calves, but what you do for them benefits the whole leg. Walking upstairs is a good thing. Not running up, you understand, or carrying all yesterday's ironing or the whole file on the Charity Ball. But a leisurely, well-postured climb is fine. You can also run in place or prance, which is really more fun because it makes you feel like a good horse — fundamental and fast. Up to fifteen prances, with your breathing keyed to your speed.

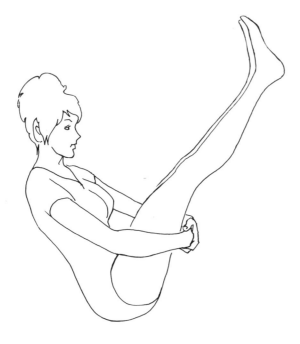

2. *For the calves:* Stand with the right foot forward, carrying most of the body weight, and with knee bent. The left leg is stretched far enough back so that the heel never touches the floor. Now lean forward and press into the right leg, then rock slightly back, so that the left heel comes down but not all the way. Relax and change legs. Eight times each leg.

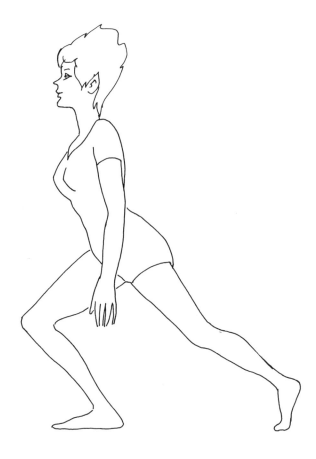

FEET AND ANKLES

Your feet should be able to look up to you, especially in summer. They are, true enough, at the bottom of the figure you have been fashioning, hopefully along the sensible lines we outline in our book. In view of the supporting role they take in your life all year round, you should give your feet special consideration in warm weather. It is truly their season in the sun.

The first thing to do is let them out.

More than any bodily extremity, the feet are confined much of the time in strong, warm materials for reasons of support, climate, or chic. If you are young, you have probably escaped the torture of the high, high heel (that forward thrust into the metatarsal arch is murder) and its concomitant punishment, the pointed toe. You may, in fact, have given up shoes altogether.

Wherever you hit the calendar, you should be

clever enough to buy what shoes you do wear in the moderate-heel range, properly fitted by someone who knows his business, to carry the constant load that is you. This does not mean shoes have to be clumpy, though the Clementine Look ("herring boxes without topses") has been with us for some time now. But the good boot, like the good suit, never departs the area of high style.

When the time finally comes for you to take off everything you can and let the fresh air get to as much of you as possible, no part of you is going to be happier than your feet. And you'd better look higher, as well. With the impending descent of the skirt, the ankle seems destined to replace the knee (again) as woman's most exciting joint.

Presumably you have been providing nominal care all year long by keeping your toenails trimmed, the cuticles oiled and pushed back, and the troublesome calluses buffed away. You have gotten hastily to the podiatrist if you are bothered — perish the thought — with corns. But the care needs to be intensified in summer. Sandals are next to barefoot and both necessarily toughen the skin, particularly on the heels and the outer sides of the feet. Keep them lubricated. Keep them cool and dry; at such times as they are not bare; for confined, warm moisture is not only uncomfortable but often the start of something not nice.

You cannot treat your feet as if they were cut off from the rest of you at midcalf. If you know anything at all about dynamics, you know that dead weight is harder to shift than distributed weight, and you will recall the points we have made about breathing, posture, tuck, and lift. Breathing is basic, whatever you do. Posture is the carriage of the body, sitting or standing or lying. Tuck is our short word for the proper position of the pelvic structure to support the load above it. Lift is that quality of stretch that nets upward and outward to keep the nonbony ingredients from huddling in unattractive places.

If you remember these points, you will help your feet. They are equipped for their job with things you can see — the incredibly graceful structure of the arch — and with things you can't see — complex network of bones, nerves, and tendons. Unless you are athletic, however, and consistently so, your feet and ankles will stiffen with age and disuse. Here are some things you can do about it.

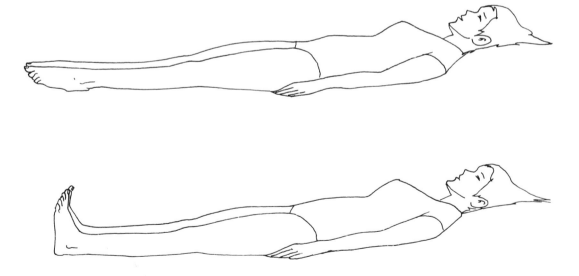

1. In bed, before you get up. Rest heels on the mattress, keep your knees stiff, point the toes directly over the arch, and curl them straight downward to the bed. Release, stretch them up toward the front of your leg. Do this sixteen times, and when you are expert, conclude each time by lifting your entire leg, stiff-kneed still, as far off the bed and up as is comfortable, from the hip. This is a bonus for your entire leg and the lower stomach muscles.

51

2. Stand in good posture and raise your body on half-toe (not as far up as tiptoe), then go back down. Sixteen times. Hold arms out to the side to balance, if you wish.

It is almost impossible to deal with toes independently in matters of exercise, which is surprising when you consider how independently important they are to your mobility. They control the walk finally — its buoyancy, its direction, its subtlety. If you don't think so, tie your feet up, each into a bundle, and try to navigate.

3. A good thing to do with toes is to scrunch them up, as if you were trying to gather them back

CHAPTER 10

"OR WOULD YOU RATHER BE
A FISH?" — WATER EXERCISES

into the feet. Then open them out, stretch wide, and count off, one by one, folding them — or trying to — back under. Begin with the little one and work toward the big toe. Eight times.

The Throwaway

Roll or circle the foot, from the ankle, with or without shoes. You are describing a wide, horizontal oval in the air with your big toe, and you should do it eight to sixteen times. It may cramp your feet at first. If it does, just flex them backward and rest a minute. Eventually, you will get to know when you need this exercise.

Your feet will tell you.

Water is a whole other world, and nowhere more so than in the area of exercise.

The heavy clarity and flow of water seem to heighten the excitement of anything that goes on in it. Its buoyancy punctuates the action. In athletic events, everything is speed and splash; in water ballets and spectacles, it is sparkle and grace. These same qualities of weight and buoyancy serve quite another function when you come into water

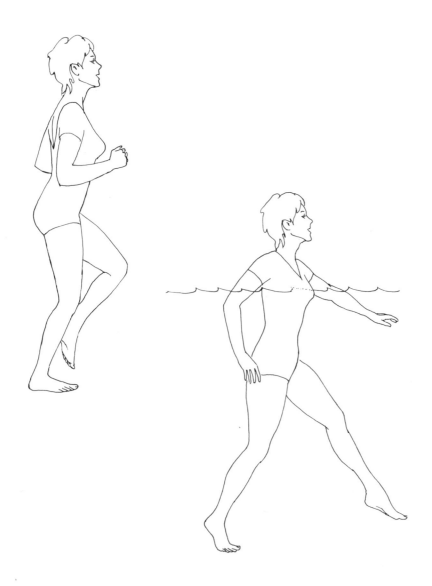

for exercise planned specifically to firm your body. You use its character to help you.

When you move against the weight of the water, its resistance does some of your work for you. The fact that your body will float does another part of the job. But you have to stay in the command post and direct the maneuver.

The difference between air and water seems obvious. The difference between how your body works in the two environments may be more subtle. If you are jumping around at the poolside, there is nothing surrounding your body to hinder you — you are dealing only with the gravity which pulls you back to earth. The resistance you meet is vertical. In breast-deep water, you seem able almost to defy gravity as you push yourself joyously upward. But your resistance is horizontal: it surrounds you. Try jogging to get an immediate idea. Do a lap around the pool (off the concrete, please), then get in the pool and try the same thing (an excellent exercise, by the way). In water, those leg muscles obey when you tell them to come up, but they are slower about getting down. It will take you a little time to get accustomed to the difference in delivery time between what you tell your body to do, in water, and how quickly it gets done. You use the time lapse to make lazy muscles work.

If you can have even a little supervised water exercise training, so much the better. Many country clubs, athletic clubs, and YM- and YWCAs have such programs. But if there are none near you — or if you just feel adventurous — then get in and find out for yourself.

What you get into is the next consideration. Private pools have multiplied vastly in the last decade, but when people talk about water exercise they nearly always mean swimming or a water-oriented sport, not the use of water in a planned program to firm the body. Pools for body exercise have, ideally, a few more requirements which you might wish to consider, if your pool is still in your future.

If you are in the planning stage, you have presumably already examined your priorities — who is to use the pool (toddlers? responsible adults? growing-and-soon-to-leave-home children?), how you are going to keep them safe in it and around it, and how you are going to maintain it. Additional points to consider are these:

a. A flat pool floor which meets the side walls at a 90-degree angle. The slope from shallow to deep won't matter so much, but it is very nearly impossible to do an exercise which depends on side-wall support, if your feet are continuously slipping out from under you on a rounded pool bottom.

b. An area along the side, at a depth of about four feet and well away from the diving board, where a bar (similar to a ballet bar) can be fastened. This provides good work space. If you are very serious, you can arrange side slots so that a temporary bar can be dropped in across the pool. It is potentially dangerous, however, and should be removed once you are through your work.

c. An underwater ledge on which to walk (since striding along in knee-deep water is a fabulous exercise) or to sit while you are doing more ambitious things. The top of the ledge should be about a foot below the surface and in a pool area where the total depth is about four feet. The water should just about reach your waist when you sit on the ledge, and your feet should be on the bottom of the pool. Let the ledge be the first level below the water surface (be careful about steps: they wave under water) and border it with a contrasting tile or other material, so that the edge is clearly defined.

d. Temperature control. If you are stalwart, you can exercise in the same temperature of water you swim in — somewhere in the 80s — provided you stop and swim a few laps when you get cold. Chill will make you tense and will destroy your whole exercise program. You need water in the low 90s for good exercising — not only is it more pleasant, but the warmth loosens the muscles and makes everything easier.

This pool equipment gives you more versatility, but you don't have to have it. You can probably work out substitutes of your own. What equipment you do have to have is fortunately simple and easily available. It is a pair of thick-walled, smooth balls. You can buy them anywhere, but they must be sturdy and they should be between eight and ten inches in diameter.

Correct breathing is vital in any water activity, and more vital — if that is possible — in exercise, simply because it provides you with a major means of control. When you inhale, you add something lighter than water to your body and you rise to the surface. When you exhale, you lessen your ability to float and you sink. So when you are trying to get the thighs to go down through persistently buoyant water, blow out your breath. Get it back when you want them up.

Here is a selection of water exercises planned for several different body areas. You may be happy to remember the bonus truth that almost anything you do with your legs in water helps tighten your stomach muscles.

1. Start with the water jog we mentioned above, but do it in place. That is, submerge your shoulders, bend your knees slightly, and hold your arms out in front. Run on the spot, touching your knees to your arms without bouncing, keeping your back straight and your pelvis tucked in. Eighty to one hundred times.

2. *Waist-twisters.* Sitting on the ledge, or steps, support yourself with your hands on the edge. Bring your bent knees to the surface and let your hips float off the ledge, but with your hands still

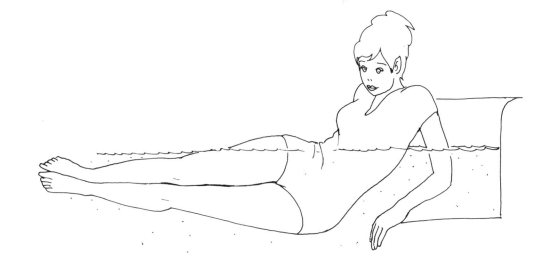

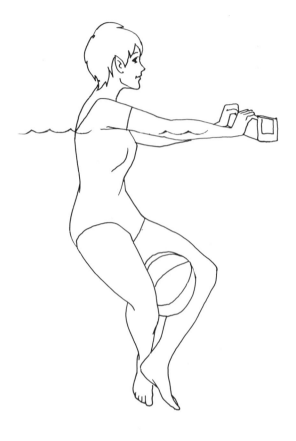

controlling you. Now, with elbows bent and shoulders relaxed, twist to one side getting your hips up as close to the surface as you can. Exhale and twist back the other way, letting the other hip come up. Feel the pull through the waist, not the shoulders. Forty to fifty times.

Waist-twister variation: Another way to do this, without the ledge, is a little more fun because a ball underwater is always unpredictable. Standing close to the bar, or the side of the pool, cross your legs at the ankles. Do a half-sit, opening your knees. Press one ball down to rest just between them, so that you can grip it with your knees. Now grasp the side of the pool and swivel first to one side, then the other, with your back straight, rather as you might have done as a child at an old-fashioned soda fountain. You can vary this exercise by keeping your knees in the sit position and bringing one hip to the surface on one side, then exhaling and bringing up the other. It is a cinch, once you stop the ball from bouncing up and smacking you in the face. Forty to fifty times.

3. *Heel clicks for the thighs.* Stand with legs wide apart, knees and toes out, and bend the knees until the shoulders are just underwater. Hold your arms out to the sides for balance, and, breathing regularly, pick up your feet and click the heels together (with toes to the sides) while your pelvis stays safely tucked and your back is straight. Don't let your body bounce; make the thigh muscles work. Thirty to forty times.

4. *For your arms, the Washboard.* Standing chest high in water, put your hands around the top of one ball, with the middle fingers touching and the elbows out. Now push the ball down under and do a 6-to-8-inch up-and-down motion in front of your stomach, close to your body, without letting the ball surface. Twenty to thirty times.

There are a series of beautiful tricks you can do with your water balls that are good for the whole lower half of your body. First, push one ball out in front of you, and, holding on to it, propel yourself with a firm flutter kick for a couple of pool lengths. The legs move up and down from the hips and the knees are relaxed but not bent. Then try a frog kick. Holding on to that ball, bring your legs in and up toward your inner thighs, the soles of your feet facing each other. Then thrust them out in a large V and bring the legs back together with the knees straight.

Now put a ball under each arm and sit down in the water, pelvis tucked and back straight, and your legs straight in front. Move backward through the water with the same flutter kick. Correct posture will keep your balance. Do the same using the frog kick. In all these exercises, you will travel through the water, but speed is not your aim. It is not where you get but what you do while you are

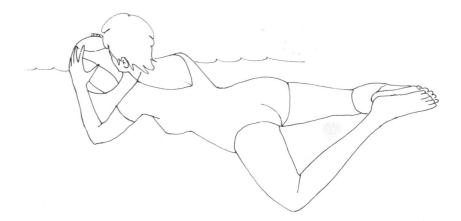

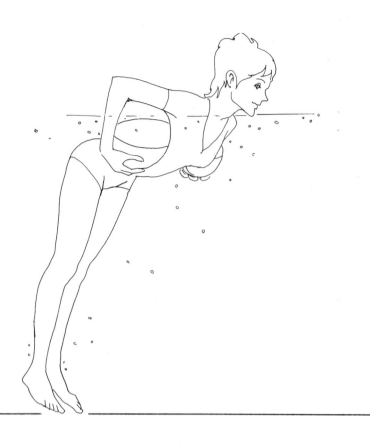

going that counts. The more water you push with your legs, the more good you do your hips and thighs.

Another beauty is the Rocking Chair, which is simple but which somehow gives a great sense of achievement when you have mastered it. Put a ball under each arm and do a half-sit in the water. Breathe in, push your elbows slowly back, and let your straight legs float up behind you. When they surface, breathe out slowly, bring your elbows forward and, holding your feet flexed and your legs still straight, let them come under you in a jack-knife until they are in front, in the straight-legged

CHAPTER 11

THE LITTLE HELPS —
MAN-MADE AIDS

half-sit from which you started. You can lollop back and forth in the water like this for fifteen to twenty times and do all kinds of good to almost everything.

In water, as in any other environment for exercise, you get results in ratio to what effort you put in. The beautiful thing about water is that the ratio is friendlier. No matter how little work you do, it produces some good. Besides, it is so much fun. Water, by its very character, gives you a feeling of litheness and grace as you move through it. On land, you have to make your movements beautiful. In water, they can't help but be.

There is an infallible truth about exercise: you do have to do it yourself. You set the goal. You pick the implements. You use them. Most of these implements are in your head — your clear knowledge of what you want to do; the program you evolve to do it; your determination to make it work.

We have generally stayed away from recommending any manual devices to help you, particularly the large, mechanical ones, though many spas and retreats do use them. They help in break-

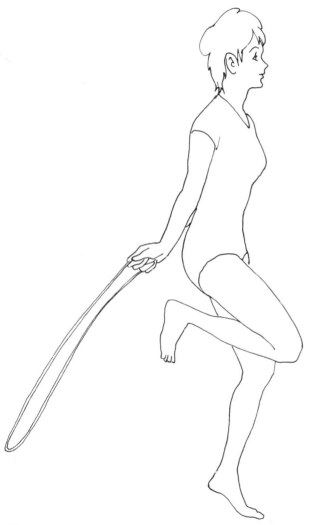

ing down tissue and can be of value in an overall program that includes individual exercise. But they cannot tone your skin or firm your body, and so if you are not careful, you may find that although you have broken down excess fat magnificently and dieted off the extra weight, you are left with a distressingly sagged carrying case.

There are, however, some simple outside aids that you may wish to use in conjunction with your own program. They include a pole, a slant board, a pair of small weights, and a jump rope. You may buy them, in lines of varying elegance and expense, at many stores, from specialty shops to supermarkets. You may even find them around your house.

The pole can be a sawed-off broomstick, or a wand of commercial manufacture, made of lightweight aluminum with tipped ends. Our only recommendation is that it be about 36 inches long, round, and light. Use it to push against in some exercises, as a balance aid in others. It is not a necessity, but it may provide variety in your routine.

Buy any kind of jump rope you please and the only exercise you need do with it is to jump it. Please don't bound up and down on two feet at a time. Use only one, but jump on it twice — once as the rope goes under and once while the rope is going over your head; then shift to the other foot. You can work up to one hundred jumps.

The slant board is a gently upholstered flat board, 18 to 20 inches in width, and about 6 feet in length.

It rests on the floor at one end and on little legs about a foot high at the other end. You rest on it, head at the lower end, legs to the higher end, and with knees slightly bent. This position is excellent for relaxation and the board is a help for some exercises. Stay off it if you have any blood pressure problems.

The board is especially good for abdominal exercises. Here are a few.

1. With your legs on the board, lie down with arms overhead on the floor. Let your breath out, and, raising your arms over and toward your knees, pull your body about a quarter of the way to a sitting position. Roll back down, breathing in. Eight times.

2. Bring the knees to the chest, holding the side of the board with the hands, and raise the right leg up to the ceiling, pressing with the heel. Lower the right leg, at the same time raising the left. Keep heel pressing and stomach pulled in. Eight times.

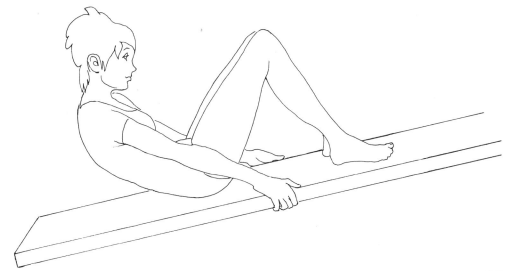

3. With hands on the sides of the board, knees apart and bent, breathe in, tuck pelvis under, and begin to roll the back up into a low arc, keeping the abdominal muscles flat. Lower back, vertebra by vertebra. Don't go too high; you get the good by going down very slowly and paying attention to the tuck.

You should not use weights at all until you are very familiar with the exercises that involve them. You may buy weights, which should be of the 3-pound variety, use empty king-size drink bottles, paperweights, grapefruits — anything that is easy to hold and feels good in your hand. They are most effective in exercises for the upper arms and back.

1. Grasp the weights so that your fingers are in front and hold your arms straight out to the sides. Do small, 12-inch circles, about one a second, then let your arms drop slowly to your sides. Repeat and work up to thirty circles.

2. Stand with a weight in each hand and bend elbows to bring hands in to the chest, legs apart and knees relaxed. Now breathe in and open the arms, letting the body bend forward from the waist as the arms move to the back as far as is comfortable (you are Anna Pavlova dancing "The Swan").

CHAPTER 12

TENSION — FINAL STATEMENT

Now tuck the pelvis to avoid back strain, and begin the return trip, bringing the arms back to the chest and straightening to a standing position. Eight times.

A plastic or vinyl exercise pad may give you some creature comfort and will not make your exercise program any less spartan. In some exercises, your neck may be more comfortable if you roll a small towel and put it underneath (not a big, furry towel — the hand-towel size is better).

Available in bath and linen shops, and more and more popular, are the small, round, tubular neck pillows. They are good for reading in bed and can help you rest with an unrestful hairdo, but most importantly they can relieve tension in the neck muscles and show you where your head should be when you are lying down.

Tension is the personality pollutant of our time.

We live in a climate charged with it. There is protest, conflict, and uncertainty on the one hand; incredible horizons of new knowledge on the other. So much good excitement and bad excitement make it very nearly impossible to stay uninvolved enough to find a life balance. Every transition age must have seemed the same to the people living in it, but it is still astounding how fast and continuously today's news travels. It seems unfair that even if we surmount our personal obstacles, we must still be bombarded by anxieties from the outside.

We are living, at the same time, in a culture where youth is overemphasized. Even though one admires the clarity and objectivity with which much of the younger generation is tracking its goals, it is hard to maintain an evenness of self-evaluation in a world whose media so often present a woman over fifty as a caricature or a stereotype.

The older woman has to do a kind of reverse pioneering to find out where she is. It does not hurt the younger one to make the same canny self-assessment. Not only are we prone to assume that our bodies will somehow always stay young; we have been led into despising them because they don't. We say, "My body isn't what it used to be." No, it is not. It is better than it used to be. It should bear the patina of the wear and care you have given it. The changes that come with age should be considered badges of service rather than signs of deterioration.

We have said that what you feel about yourself is reflected in your posture, your carriage, and your presence. You must value yourself, but with an amused tolerance for your own shortcomings. This is the balance you aim for, and tension can destroy it almost as surely as disease. Tension is, in fact, a disease, and while we wouldn't presume to deal with it medically, we have certainly tried to show you how to deal with it physically.

The best thing to do about tension is to stand up to it, literally. The implications of outside problems scale down as you get better control of your own. The simple act of straightening your body is a good health habit and a psychological peg. You are expressing outside what you are feeling inside — maybe before you feel it. But as you train yourself to sit well and stand well, the sense of lightness and lift comes automatically. At the same time, you must fight another enemy — gravity. It is a sad truth that the major problems of the maturing figure have a tendency to settle into each other between the shoulders and thighs. Good posture halts the trend.

The best posture exercise is still the basic roll-down-and-up included in the Ten-Minutes-a-Day Program for Fitness from *Fashion Your Figure*. You have gotten out of bed with your body folded at the waist, arms down and loose. Now wind yourself up the spine, tucking in your buttocks and lifting your torso so that you cannot help but come into an easy and correct standing position.

If posture is the starting signal, resiliency is certainly the goal. You are born with beautiful muscle tone, and it will maintain itself under normal con-

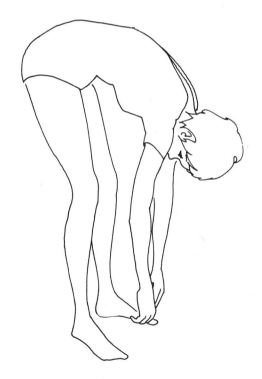

ditions until you are about twenty-five. Then it begins to need help. You ought to start giving that help in your teens — primarily to establish the habit, but also to correct errors of posture and carriage. Tone will come back with good and consistent exercise programs, but it is considerably harder to regain if you wait to start until you are in your midforties.

The basic program we mention is a good starting point, and the philosophy behind it is not complicated. Good movement produces well-being and well-being is the impetus to continuing good movement. This program, used and tailored to your own requirements, will fight a good battle against tension. But for extra skirmishes:

1. Sitting in good posture and looking straight ahead, bounce your shoulders in a fast up-and-down eight times. Go lax. Then repeat eight times.

Variation: Lift your shoulders forward into your

neck, then circle them back up and to the neck again. Repeat full circle eight times and relax.

2. Sitting, drop the head until your chin touches your chest in the center. Keeping the chin in, slowly turn the face up to the right as far as it will go comfortably. Then slowly turn it back down to center and then up to left. Eight complete half-circles, and don't hurry. That slow-down warning holds for any exercise that involves the neck.

3. Sitting, let the face and head relax onto the chest, mouth open and jaws loose. Wind the back down, arms down to the side, until your head is in your lap. Stay there for a count of ten and then roll yourself back up. Repeat eight times.

Your personal rhythms are always with you. Listen to your heartbeat. Listen to your breathing: hopefully in long, beautiful, and calm breaths. Listen to the quiet in your spirit, and don't let the outside world jam your personal frequency.